10 Essential Oils
You Must Have

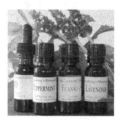

The most powerful oils and
blends and how to use them

GAIL THACKRAY

Printed in the United States of America

Thackray, Gail

10 essential Oils You Must Have

Layout and design and cover art by Teagarden Designs

ISBN: 978-1-948358-06-4

Published by
Lady of Light
Indian Springs Publishing
P.O. Box 286
La Cañada, CA 91012
www.indianspringspublishing.com

CONTENTS

INTRODUCTION TO OILS & ELIXIRS

Natural Essential Oils, tincture, essences and homeopathic remedies are becoming more and more popular as people learn that they are not only much more effective than many western medicine treatments, they usually have little, if any negative side-effects. In fact, they have been used very effectively and safely for centuries.

Oils and tinctures work physically on our body and often bring fast, visible results. But they are not only working on a physical level, in fact they work so well because they change the underlying energy vibration of our own life force frequency, removing blocks that are causing us health issues. But oils can also be used to affect our energy in many other ways, such as to deepen our intuition, strengthen our energy, lift our mood and even draw to us the things that we desire.

Vibrational Essences or Flower Essences are different from essential oils. The oil is the actual physical oil from the flower or plant. An essence is the energetic imprint of the flower or plant. It is obtained with a very tiny amount of the flower, plant or even crystal or sacred object, infused into distilled or blessed water in a similar way to a homeopathic remedy. The oil is the actual physical evidence of the plant, often thought as being the energy of the plant. Oils are very concentrated and often have a strong distinctive taste and smell. Flower essence is a spiritual imprint or vibration of the plant which may have very little taste or smell. Some people may prefer one to the other and oils and essences can also be combined very effectively. I will mostly concentrate on essential oils, but I will also discuss a few essences that are worth considering.

To learn which oils to choose, how to blend oils, and how to most effectively use them, can be a life long study, but I have chosen to focus on some of the most significant ones, for some of the common uses you may have. Most importantly, I will show you how to test which ones are most suited to your personal energy for the result you are looking for.

I have listed some remedies and uses of essential oils and although essential oils are very safe, and very few people ever report any negative side-effects, you should always consult your doctor if you have any health concerns or to see if the use of any of these treatments are right for you. This information is meant to help you with your search for optimal health and vitality and should not be considered an alternative to medical advice and care.

Ancient Oils

The incorporation of essential oils and tinctures into daily life, dates back many centuries with evidence of their extensive use from ancient Egyptian times, to biblical days, to the more recent herbalists of the sixteenth and seventeenth centuries. Some oils were so potent, the practitioners were sometimes said to be magicians and sometimes accused of witchcraft. But oils and elixirs are thought to date even further back to the days of Lemuria and Atlantis. Now these secrets have been recently revealed in ancient documents as well as channeled, through mediums and psychics who receive messages from guides and masters in spirit. Edgar Cayce is a wonderful example of a modern-day prophet who through trance, was said to have been given many details of oils and their uses from guides in spirit. Much of this is ancient knowledge that is only recently resurfacing and being revisited.

Many people with a passion and an instinct for essential oils have hidden knowledge from past-lives. For those people, it will feel like a remembrance of this knowledge. However, sometimes there can be an unconscious fear because the person was persecuted in the past, perhaps for working with herbs and tinctures and being accused of practicing medicine without a license or doing witchcraft. Today that person may have a subconscious fear of working with oils or making the wrong decision. If this is the case, doing intuition meditations with the oils will help to reconnect you with their inner secrets and release any fears and blocks you may have.

Grade & Quality

There is a big difference in the quality of oils on the market. You need to look for not only organically grown but the best oils are from very carefully selected crops, harvested at the right time of the year and even under the optimum astrological influences. Most importantly is the process by which the oils are extracted and prepared. And of course, make sure your essential oil is pure or a blend of pure oils. A high-quality oil will not need any additives. Be aware of any "filler" oils, or "carrier" oils or preservatives which could dilute and diminish the properties.

The grade and process of the oils that you choose is of upmost importance. Several oils and remedies are best if the oil is taken orally. For this it is necessary that you choose an ingestible grade oil. Even for those used topically, you are still absorbing them into your blood stream and therefore you really need ingestible grade oils. For oils that can be used in a room, in ceremonies or in a diffuser, the grade is not as important, however it is always safer to go with a high-grade oil.

I found an organic farmer, who not only prepares the oils for the highest quality, but is also a Reiki Master, and does Reiki on the crops regularly. Additionally, the crops are arranged and grown in accordance to Feng Shui. When I tuned into the energy of the land, I found that the area was a vortex of high spiritual energy and very connected to Pleiadean beings, like the energy of crop circles. Funnily enough the farmer reported sightings regularly on the farm.

I am working with this grower to use John of God blessed water and crystal energy in the preparation, as well as sacred oils from other amazing healers around the world. I then infuse them myself to encode them with high spiritual vibrations for the desired purpose.

Oils will usually come in cobalt blue glass to protect them from the harmful rays of the sun and to avoid the formation of unwanted compounds. Molecules may leach from a plastic container and react with the oil producing impurities. Store your oils in a cool pantry or place in the house. They do not need to be refrigerated but they should not be left out in bright sunlight. They can keep their energy for a year or more if they are stored correctly. This is more important for the oils you plan to ingest. If the date is questionable, no need to throw them away, you can use these in your diffusers and in ceremonies.

Many essential oils are preserved with alcohol or contain filler oil. The oils and blends I would recommend are pure essential oils with no fillers or alcohol. You can always add your essential oil to almond oil or olive oil for massage or topical use but if the bottle already includes these oils then the actual essential oil you are getting is very diluted and these are probably not ingestible grade oils.

Essences are usually preserved with alcohol. It is better to find ones preserved with a tiny amount of atomic Iodine (as prescribed by Edgar Cayce in his trance readings). These contain Iodine Tricloride (not from shell fish which some people can be allergic to). I have not found anyone to be allergic to these essences even those with shell fish allergies. This also makes these a source of Iodine.

HOW TO USE OILS & ELIXIRS

Orally

Several oils and remedies are best if the oil is taken orally. For this make sure the oil is absolutely an ingestible grade. For ingestible oils, you can add them to a glass of water. It is important to use glass or ceramic, not plastic. If the oils are a concentrated high-grade oil, it can dissolve the plastic and then you would end up drinking plastic which would not be good. For most oils about 4 drops in a glass of water is good. You can muscle test if you need more. Generally, 3-4 drops would be normal, 10 drops would be high dose for a strong or difficult issue and 1-2 drops would be a low or maintenance dose. Additional drops are not going to harm you, but it may be wasting the extra drops.

Alternatively, you can place the drops directly in the mouth, by putting a few drops under the tongue. The part of the mouth under the tongue is very absorbent and this allows the oil to get into the blood stream quickly. Be sure not to touch the dropper with your tongue so as not to contaminate the rest of the oil.

Another way to ingest is to place a few drops on the back of your hand and lick your hand. You may find some oils too strong or the taste undesirable to put directly in the mouth and prefer to add to water which is perfectly fine.

Sprays are usually a little less concentrated and you can spray them under your tongue. In the case of a sore throat, spray directly at the back of the throat.

Inhale

To inhale you can run a few drops between your palms and then cup your hands over your nose and mouth and take deep inhaling breaths. It will dissipate quickly, so you may need to repeat this several times. You can also place the bottle directly under your nose and keep inhaling. If some oils touch your nose, they may burn or sting a little.

Diffuse

You can use a room diffuser to put the oil in a vapor throughout the room. Steam diffusers are made for this purpose and usually they are electric. You will place a few drops of oil in the water, as instructed. If you have a steam-room or sauna, the oils can be placed either directly over the steam outlet or in an open container inside the steam room to fill the room with the vapor.

Other types of diffusers may include burners. This is a glass or ceramic mini bowl which holds a small amount of the oil and usually hangs over a candle flame. The flame heats up the container and the oil evaporates into the room.

You can make your own personal steamer which is great for colds or flu and can be used to inhale other essential oils. To make a personal steamer, boil a pan of water. Place the pan of hot water on a table or floor where you can easily lean your face over it. Add a few drops of oil into the still hot water. Place your face above the steam and the vapors and cover your head and the whole pan in a thin cloth or bed sheet. You will need to quickly place your face over the pan and cover with a cloth, because as soon as you add the drops of oil, the vapor will dissipate quickly.

It is great to always use high grade oils, even with the diffusers but if you have a lesser quality oil, you can safely use these in your room diffuser.

Spray Aura

Oils, essences and tinctures sometimes come in the form of sprays. These can be sprayed around your aura. Especially spray over the top of the crown and in a halo pattern over the top of the head.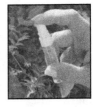

They can also be sprayed directly on an object for cleansing, such as when cleansing a crystal. In the case of cleansing a crystal, spray directly on the point of the crystal as this is where the energy concentrates.

Topical

Oils can be placed directly on the skin, temples or forehead. For example, the Egyptian Moringa oil should be rubbed on the face and under the eyes as a face cream and to remove wrinkles. Peppermint can be rubbed on the temples for a headache or onto a part of the body where there is pain. Geranium-rose oil can be rubbed on the third eye (between the eyes in the center of the forehead) to increase intuition and mediumship.

When rubbing an oil on the third eye, or heart chakra, you are enhancing the power, so you want to rub in a clockwise direction at the same time holding your intent. If you wanted to diminish something, such as a blemish, rub the oil in a counter-clockwise direction.

Bathing in essential oil is another way to use the oil topically. Add about 10 drops to your bathwater or salt scrub. You can use several oils and mixing the oils does not have any adverse effects.

You can also add a few drops of oil into a massage oil or body lotion.

For topical use on the skin, it is important to use a good grade ingestible quality oil. Even though you are not ingesting it, our skin is the largest organ of our bodies and does absorb the oil directly into our blood stream.

There are some practices that advocate putting several essential oils concentrated directly onto the skin. For most areas of the body, this can be too strong. For over-all massage, I recommend diluting several drops into olive oil, almond oil or coconut oil. It is good to use the concentrated oil on a burn or ailment or on the third eye or temples, however for a large or sensitive area of the body diluting with a body oil would be recommended.

An essential oil wrap is a wonderful way to infuse the oils into your body. First add a few drops of essential oils into almond oil or olive oil. Then cover the body with this oil. Then have a friend wrap you in warm moist towels. You can then be wrapped in a Mylar blanket and either wrapped in warm blankets or preferably on a heating pad. You can also do a dry wrap by placing the essential oils on your chakras and lie on a heating pad covered with a Mylar blanket. I'll talk more on Baths and Wraps at the end of this book.

Ceremonies

Oils can be rubbed directly on an item for anointment, such as on a candle or statue or on a photo. If you are using an oil on a candle to empower something, you should rub around the candle in a clock-wise motion. If you wish to diminish something, such as releasing an ailment or a negative condition, rub the oil around the candle in a counter-clockwise direction.

If you make your own candles, the oils can be added to the actual candle wax. Be very careful when working with hot candle wax and oils as they can be very flammable. This is only recommended for people who are experienced at this.

Oils can be used for burning in a fire offering. Oils may be placed inside a metal dish or on some silver-foil would also work. They can also be used to dip sage, incense or Palos Santos wood. Again, be careful if working with fire and make sure the oils do not make the item extremely flammable.

Oils can be used for protection and can be rubbed directly onto an object or an area of a room or a piece of furniture such as a chair.

A Reiki Master or other healer may use essential oils in an attunement process where they place a drop of oil on their recipient's chakras to anoint the student as they touch their student's chakras and palms. A Reiki healer can also put oil in their hands to enhance the energy flow. Oils can be used on clients during a massage, however you should always ask your client their permission and always use organic high-grade oil on a person's skin.

If you are using an oil to burn, rub on an object or rub in the corners of the room, you can use a lesser grade oil or an oil that you are not sure is good enough for ingesting.

IMPORTANT ESSENTIAL OILS & BLENDS

I am often asked what are the main essential oils that I use regularly. I am sharing the ones I absolutely love and always keep on-hand and some important blends of oils that I have, ready-made. In addition, I am including a few other sprays, ointments and tinctures that I believe are ones that are very useful to have.

These are my top 10 favorites, my everyday "must have" list:

- Geranium-Rose
- Lavender
- Eucalyptus
- Peppermint
- Frankincense
- Egyptian Oil
- Immune Support Blend
- Respiratory Blend
- Weight Loss Blend
- Throat Soothe Blend

Geranium-Rose

Intuition

A mix of Geranium and Rose oils. This is a very high frequency blend that lifts your vibration and helps you to get in the higher realms where you can connect with your guides and Angels. It surrounds you with love and protection.

This is great for mediumship and connecting with guides. Rub a few drops in your palms and inhale deeply a few times. Then rub a few drops on your third eye in a clockwise motion. This allows for deeper meditation and visions. It allows messages to flow to you. It also brings peace and wisdom and helps you to relax and stop "trying" too hard, which would prevent the psychic flow.

Edgar Cayce, through his trace readings recommended a body and face oil that included Rose Oil, mixed with Peanut and Almond Oils.

The Rose Oil also calls in the protection of Mother Mary and so can be used to protect your energy body as well as for ceremonies.

This one smells wonderful and can be used as a perfume! If used around the room, it draws in angels and guides to the room.

This also draws a wonderful connection between mother and daughter and so is a great gift to mom, grandma, aunt or daughter.

Lavender

Relaxation

Known to reduce stress, lower blood pressure and aid with relaxation and sleep. Rub a few drops on your temples when you need to relax or have a hard time sleeping. You can also put a diffuser with Lavender Oil by your bed or spray a few drops onto your pillow.

It is also wonderful for skin irritations, blemishes or allergies. For skin ailments rub a few drops directly on the area. Lavender is a great oil to have on hand in case of stings, bug bites and burns. Often this reduces the pain and swelling almost instantly.

It is known to affect the female hormones, especially estrogen. There is a lot of controversy as to whether it increases or balances this hormone. Most research suggests that it balances either a lack or an excess of estrogen. You can rub on your abdomen or you can ingest if you like the taste.

For those of you that are clairsentient this is a must as it dissolves anxiety and allergies that are caused by other people's energies you may have taken on.

Mice, ants and other bugs don't like Lavender or Peppermint, so placing a few drops around your house or in a diffuser, is a great natural way to keep them away. Dogs and cats however love Lavender Oil and it is very relaxing and balancing for them.

Eucalyptus

Psychic Detox
Eucalyptus cleanses the body both physically and spiritually, removing negative energies. You can add a few drops in your massage oil or body oil or you can put about 10 drops in your bath water for a detox bath.

It is known to help with respiratory issues and is a great oil to use if you have a flu, cold or a stuffy nose. It helps to release congestion and cleanse the lungs and chest. Use in a diffuser or steam shower to inhale. This is great to use in a personal diffuser. To make a personal diffuser, boil a pan of water, then lift it off the stove to a place where you can put it and lean over safely. Then add a few drops of oil and lean over covering your head with a thin cloth to keep as much steam in as possible as you inhale the vapors. The vapor may be very strong at first, so be careful, but it quickly evaporates, so you may have to repeat several times. Or you can put a few drops in your palms and inhale. It will be too strong to put on your skin directly under your nose, but you can try on your chest. You can also hold the bottle under your nose and inhale the vapors.

Eucalyptus is also great for energizing. Use in a body oil or in a bath to cleanse your aura and give you more energy. If it is in a room, it will lift the energy of the room.

Eucalyptus also brings courage and confidence.

This resonates with and can draw Native American guides.

Peppermint

Uplift Spirit
Peppermint is great to give you that pep in your step if you need a quick energizer. It elevates mood as it releases trapped

emotional energies. A few drops on your tongue or inhaled from your palms will lift your spirit.

It also works great on pain on the physical level. If you have a headache, place a few drops directly on your headache, your third eye and temples and this almost always instantly clears your head. Peppermint is good for other aches and pains. You can rub it directly on the area that hurts but also place it on your temples. This is because it is releasing the emotional blocks in your energy field that can cause physical pain.

It can be used in drinks and deserts and of course it can be used as a much healthier alternative to breath mint!

A few drops in a glass of water in the morning will help to get you awake and give you energy for the day.

Mice and bugs don't like Lavender or Peppermint, so placing a few drops around your house or in a diffuser, is a great natural way to keep them away.

Frankincense

Christ Consciousness

Frankincense was presented by The Wise Men to Jesus because it was revered as one of the most precious oils of the time. Frankincense resin was used during ceremonies and prayer throughout the temple and to anoint the altar. It was expensive even in those days and therefore it was significant that they would bring it as a present to baby Jesus. It was a sign that they believed he was someone of importance.

Having magical powers and miraculous healing properties, Frankincense was used for curing many ailments. It draws in the Chris Consciousness and often a smell of Frankincense will appear spontaneously during high spiritual connection.

The scent of Frankincense is often associated with the presence of Jesus. When I did dome filming of the icon of Jesus that weeps oil there was a strong smell of both Frankincense and Rose. When the prayers were about Jesus we could distinctly smell Frankincense. When the prayers were about Mary we could smell roses. The icon painting did weep oil in noticeable amounts.

Frankincense is known as an antibacterial and antiviral agent and can be used on the skin or taken internally if it is ingestible grade. You can place it on cuts and scrapes or any place on the body that needs healing. It is one of the best ointments for the gums and can be rubbed directly in the mouth or a few drops placed on your toothbrush before your toothpaste.

You can also use a few drops on your altar or on a candle at any time you wish to bring in the Christ Consciousness. Even if you are not Christian this oil will bring in the presence and essence of Jesus. Great to use in healing and any petitions to spirit. This is a beautiful present for anyone celebrating Christmas and for bringing in the Christ energy.

It is a wonderful oil for protection and can be rubbed around a room or burned in an oil burner to lift negative energies from a room or space.

Egyptian Oil

Magic & Youth

Moringa Oliefera is the Egyptian oil known for rejuvenation. It is amazing for the face and skin. You can rub it directly on your skin as a face moisturizer, especially as a night moisturizer. It is really wonderful for removing dark eye circles or blemishes. At night before you go to sleep, rub it directly under your eyes or on your dark spots and blemishes.

This is a soothing non-irritating oil and so it can be used over the entire body. However, it would be quite expensive to use it as a body lotion, so it could be extended by mixing with a body oil.

For those of you who've had past lives in Egypt this is a very powerful oil for reconnecting you with your ancient wisdom. Rub a few drops over your third eye and heart to connect you with the magical powers of ancient Egypt. This is especially wonderful for past life work and brings about powerful visions through meditation and dreams.

Immune Support Blend

Balance
This is a great blend you can use daily to keep your auric system balanced. It contains cinnamon, cloves, eucalyptus, lemon, rosemary, thyme. Use 2-3 drops daily in a glass of water in the morning, or on the tongue to keep your immune system strong. If you are feeling particularly tired or drained, repeat this several times a day. At the first signs of a cold, flu or other infection, take about 10 drops in a glass of water and repeat several times through the day. If you have a flu or runny nose, add the Respiratory Blend as well.

Immune Support works on the physical body as well as the emotional and karmic layers. If you are doing psychic work and feel yourself drained this is a great one to keep you strong. Take a few drops in a glass of water before doing readings so your energy field is more protected.

For immune disorders take up to 10 drops a day in a glass of water each morning, until you start to feel stronger and can gradually reduce the amount of drops to about 2-3 a day.

Respiratory Blend

Clears lungs and chest
This is one of the most important emergency blends you should keep on hand. At the first signs of a hoarse throat, dry throat, sore throat, stuffy nose, flu or other cold symptoms you can use this. You can put a few drops in a glass of water or use a few drops directly on the tongue. It contains clove, eucalyptus, ginger, juniper, and peppermint oils. It is quite strong so most recommend putting this in water, but honestly, I take it straight. If you take this straight, you may want to follow this with a spoon of honey (preferably Manuka Honey). The Manuka honey is also great for cold and flu symptoms and takes away the burn from the Respiratory Blend if you put it in your mouth undiluted. You can take up to 10 drops each time, several times a day until you feel you have knocked it out.

You can also inhale by placing a few drops in your hands. This is another great one to inhale by making a personal diffuser. You can mix Eucalyptus Oil in the same personal diffuser. If you have achy flu symptoms, also add the Immune Support as well (ingest).

The Respiratory Blend opens the throat chakra as well so if you need support here you can use this more often to aid with throat, nose, mouth and gums as well as clairaudient messages from spirit. On an energetic level, it helps to "get something off your chest." If you are holding onto something you need to share, this will help you share it in the best way possible.

Weight Loss Blend

Psychic Cleanse

We gain unwanted weight because of holding onto negative thoughts, emotions, guilt and fear. The largest culprit for excess weight is carrying emotional blocks from relationships (family and x-romantic relationships). If the weight gain is mostly around the hips and thighs, then this is often related to old hurt feelings from family. We also gain weight from taking on other people's thoughts and feelings, being empathic or clairsentient. This oil blend works on the emotional psychic energy disturbances as well as the physical body so that it does not return.

It contains dill, geranium, grapefruit, juniper, lemon, peppermint oils. This blend of oils works on both the physical release and the emotional release. The oils of citrus fruits contained here are known to dissolve fat cells, but this special blend also works on the emotional layers.

Take 4-6 drops before meals in a glass of water (do not use a plastic drinking glass as it may dissolve the plastic).

This will reduce your appetite as well as enable you to burn fat cells.

Throat Soothe Blend

Throat Chakra

At the first signs of a hoarse throat, dry throat or sore throat, this is great to use. It includes Oregano Oil as well as other germicides and throat soothing agents. This can be added to a glass of water and ingested. I find it the strongest is to place a few drops or spray it directly into the back of the mouth and onto the area of the throat that hurts. You can follow this with a spoonful of Manuka Honey which is also wonderfully soothing and healing for sore throats.

Sore throats usually come from not talking to someone. Meditate on who you need to talk to and what you need to say.

This also helps with other issues of the throat chakra such as thyroid issues and problems with the gums and teeth.

For a sudden sore throat use a few drops (directly on the throat (if you can bear it) several times a day until you feel you have beat this. If it is an ongoing issue, then use 2-4 drops daily in a glass of water.

OTHER IMPORTANT OILS & ELIXIRS

In addition to the main essential oils and blends, there are some specific tinctures, sprays and oils I would like to mention.

- Ormus Gold
- Third Eye Opener
- Magnesium Oil
- Colloidal Silver
- CBD Oil
- Manuka Honey
- Blended Sprays

- All Clear Spray
- Crystal Clear Spray
- Prosperity Spray
- Attracting Love Spray
- Pet Balancing Spray

Ormus Gold

Ormus is a compound mixture of minerals. It was discovered in 1975 by an Arizona farmer, David Hudson who noticed this compound in the soil that in the sunlight literally disappeared in a flash of light. When it was tested known minerals, such as gold, iron and calcium were derived but the remaining 95% consisted of other elements not found on the periodic table. This mixture of elements appears to bring great healing, expansion of the aura and a sense of wellbeing. What Hudson really witnessed was when this material was placed in the sunlight it became one with the light and was transformed to another dimension, when it dried out it literally came back as a substance. Hudson then spent years of his life researching this substance and found that our brains contain at least 5% Ormus. These mysterious elements in Ormus have not been "scientifically discovered" yet.

It is a natural compound usually prepared from purified sea water. The one I recommend contains both sea water and John of God blessed water. It is most often used as a supplement, either orally or topically and has no reported adverse side-effects.

It contains essential minerals associated with the development of the consciousness and life force energy itself. It is thought to greatly increase intuition and can produce profound effects during meditation and mediumship sessions. Ormus is thought to help with transformation of a person on a spiritual level and to aid healing in all dimensions. Many people report when using this regularly and before meditations it greatly increases their psychic awareness as well as brings a sense of wellbeing and peace. Some of the benefits reported from using Ormus are:

- Increased psychic abilities
- Aids deeper and more vivid meditation
- Opening of the third eye and increasing visual messages
- Aids sleep, quality of sleep and lucid dreaming
- Anti-aging and regenerates cell growth
- Draws out calcium build up when applied topically

- Helps the body to hydrate
- Increases energy and a sense of well being
- Gives a sense of peace and tranquility
- Reduces aches and pains
- Reduces allergies
- Protects the aura from negative energies

Third Eye Opener

This contains coriander, elemi, frankincense, rose and sandalwood oils. This blend of oils and essences helps to clear the third eye and enable it to open, allowing clairvoyant experiences. Our third eye is associated with the Pineal Gland which over time can become clouded or calcified with a film of heavy metals from environmental toxins (most often fluoride and chlorine in our water). This blend of essential oils, minerals and flower essences helps to draw and decalcify the third eye. It removes both physical and spiritual blocks that are clouding your clairvoyance. Put a few drops on the third eye between your brows but a little higher in the center of your forehead and massage in a clockwise direction (from your left side to right) I have one that comes in a roll on that you can roll onto the third eye. Do this several times a day especially before doing psychic work.

Magnesium Oil

Most people are severely deficient in magnesium which is vital for the nerves and muscles. Low magnesium can make you more prone to migraines, headaches, muscle cramps and heart irregularities. Magnesium supplements taken orally are not easily absorbed by the body and can cause digestive issues. Topical Magnesium Oil is a great solution. This can be sprayed on the soles of the feet where it is absorbed into the system easily and quickly. If you can find magnesium oil spray mixed with Helichrysum the Helichrysum will enable the magnesium to be absorbed more easily.

Magnesium spray is great for muscle cramps and joint pain. It also brings relaxation and sleep, so it is wonderful for insomnia. It has been used to treat many other ailments including; ADHD, anxiety, chronic fatigue, Lyme, fibromyalgia, diabetes, kidney stones, osteoporosis, PMS, altitude sickness, incontinence, restless leg syndrome, asthma, hayfever, MS. It is also used for preventing hearing loss and for increasing energy and endurance.

On a Spiritual level it is removing toxic spiritual interference from negativity or jealousy and even entity attachments.

It is best to take this at night as it promotes sleep. Right before you go to bed, make sure the soles of your feet are clean and spray the oil on to your feet in bed so that you don't walk on them right after.

Colloidal Silver

Colloidal Silver has been used for thousands of years as a germicide to kill bacteria, viruses and fungus (yeast & molds). What is lesser known is it also helps psychic communication, messaging & channeling. Colloidal Silver is a solution of tiny particles of real silver in a water solution.

It has been used as a natural remedy and immune strengthener for centuries. In fact, years ago, a baby of high standing would be termed "born with a silver spoon in their mouth." This was because they would actually place a silver spoon in the baby's mouth as they knew the silver particles would protect the baby from disease.

Use a few drops of colloidal silver in the throat or under the tongue at the first sign of a cold and it really works well to ward off the flu and stop sore throats. No need to dilute in water, it is already diluted.

It is great to help the body recover from a bacterial infection or virus. Colloidal Silver naturally allows the physical body's own immune system to fight off, to cleanse, and release. Colloidal Silver is allopathic meaning that Colloidal Silver is all inclusive and can heal within the physical body most anything! You can use it every day to strengthen the immune system. 2-4 drops a day, or one spray is great for on-going use. 10 drops (3 sprays), 3-4 times a day should be used for fighting off an infection.

There is another unique use for it. When I first started as a medium I noticed that I would be drained of iron. This is because the messages from spirit are formed in a different way from normal thoughts. I discovered that spirit would use my mind and my brain synapses to form messages. This requires a tremendous amount of iron. Just a short but deep connection would deplete my iron. I was given the message from spirit that they could use silver particles just as well if not better. I tried a few drops before spirit communication and it works perfectly. In fact, it helps to make the messages clearer. Now I always use a few drops of colloidal silver before doing spirit communication or deep meditation.

Colloidal silver is also great for clearing off negative energies that you might have picked up. For this it is still recommended that you take it orally, rather than as a spray.

You can make colloidal silver with a silver ion machine. You place the negative and positive silver prongs in distilled water and leave it plugged in over-night. Small amounts of silver are electronically deposited into the water.

I have batches made with blessed John of God water. This I feel is very special because not only does it have the properties from the colloidal silver but also from the blessed water. You want to look for one with nano particles.

Colloidal Silver does not damage the tissues or interact with other medications. It is safe and wonderful to use with children and animals. Nano-particle Colloidal Silver is designed to be used on a regular basis to strengthen, repair and regenerate your immune system.

Colloidal Silver can be sprayed on the back of the throat, but you should not eat or drink or use any other oil orally for 15 minutes before and after the Colloidal Silver. Other food or liquid may dilute it and would render the Colloidal Silver ineffective.

Some people have reported turning blue from excessive use of Colloidal Silver, however these people were drinking a full glass or even a gallon of Colloidal Silver a day. 10 drops even several times a day should not cause this. Colloidal Silver should be stored in a cobalt blue glass bottle to avoid the formation of unwanted compounds (Colloidal Silver made using distilled water may leech molecules from a plastic container which could react with the silver colloid).

CBD Oil

CBD oil is an organic Cannabidol extract from the hemp or marijuana plant. It has many healing properties but because it does not contain any THC it does not make you "high." It is very important to make sure it is from an organic grower. CBD oil is usually sold in the form of an oil or tincture and the actual amount of cannabidol is usually listed, so note the strength of cannabidol per fluid ounce of oil.

A regular or maintenance dose would be 2-3 drops daily, usually in the morning, directly in the mouth or in a glass of water. If you have a strong health condition, you should try up to 10 drops three times a day. If your body does not need this much, it will not be harmful, the drops not used by the body will be flushed away. CBD can also be purchased in creams and topical lotions, if you prefer not to ingest. Creams are also good to rub on areas of the body where you may have a problem. It is also a great facial skin cream, with many reporting it rejuvenates the skin and diminishes wrinkles.

CBD was controversial for a while, however it is now legal in all States regardless of the state marijuana laws as it is not considered a "marijuana drug." The endocannabinoid system is part of an extensive network of receptors in the brain and central nervous system that help regulate the body's balance or homeostasis. Cannabinoids may affect mood, sleep, appetite, hormone regulation, pain and immune response.

CBD oil has been reported to help with:

- Pain and Inflammation
- Antipsychotic Effects
- Reducing Anxiety
- Helping to Manage Cancer
- Relieving Nausea
- Seizures and Other Neurological Disorders
- Cardiovascular Health
- Diabetes
- And for other suggested benefits to people and animals

Manuka Honey

Manuka Honey is worth mentioning here even though it is not an oil or elixir. This type of honey mostly comes from New Zealand. It is made by bees who take pollen from the Tea Trees. Tea Tree Oil is a very powerful germicide essential oil that can be used on cuts, sores and even taken internally. Manuka Honey has all the same properties of Tea Tree Oil being a wonderful germicide with the additional health benefits of this honey. It usually comes with a strength marked, such as 5+, 10+, 20+. Try to get one that has a 10+ strength or higher. You can eat this as delicious honey and it can also be placed topically on the skin. It is particularly useful for eye infections or areas of sensitive skin. You will need to test this carefully, but most people can tolerate this honey on sensitive areas.

Blended Sprays

Blended sprays can be essential oils or essences. The ones I recommend are a combination of flower or vibrational essences, essential oils and blessed water. They are unscented infusions of the energies of a particular flower, crystal, color, symbol, seed, metal, fruit or combinations of these and other organic elements. They are believed to release energy patterns and blockages at the root level.

Mists are designed to release the patterns in our energy field or aura, that cause limitation in our experience.

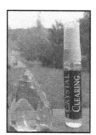

The ones I recommend have a small amount of detoxified iodine instead of alcohol.

All Clear Spray

This contains grapefruit, lime, rosemary and ylang oils and this combination of essences and oils to release negative energies from your aura. It contains sage, salt, Palos Santos, crystal energy and blessed water. All elements to cleanse you of other people's energies that you may have picked up and releases negative energy from around you. It also sets up a protection shield to stop you taking on any more negative energy. This is a great alternative to smudging with sage in a place where this is not convenient.

Crystal Clear Spray

Associated Crystals should be cleared and cleansed at least every 21 days, or more often if they are being used. If you are working on clients, using crystals, they should be cleared between sessions. This can be done with salt water, blessed water or sage. The Crystal Clear Spray is a great quick alternative to clear your crystals. It contains cardamom, clove, lemongrass and nutmeg. Spray on the points of your crystals and your crystal pendants. If others have been handling your crystals this is a great quick way to clear energy of others. It will not affect any blessing or empowerment infused in the crystal.

Prosperity Spray

This is combination of essences and oils known to draw abundance and success as well as confidence and strength. It includes cardamom, cedarwood, cinnamon, cloves and vetiver. This spray helps to remove and cleanse any blocks of lack or other issues that are holding you back. It contains flower essences and high vibrational crystal energies and blessed water. Spray this above your head, and in your aura. Especially use this before an important meeting or phone conversation.

Attracting Love Spray

This is a combination of flower essences and oils known to draw love, romance and a person's twin flame. It includes Basil, cinnamon, guaiac wood, lemongrass, spearmint and ylang oils. This spray helps to remove and cleanse old relationships to allow new ones to flourish. It contains flower essences and high vibrational crystal energies and blessed water. This is best sprayed over your head in your aura and around your sacral chakra (just below the navel).

Pet Balancing Spray

Pets respond well to energy healing and essences. This is combination of essences and oils known to remove any negative energies that pets have picked up in their environment or healing their "owners." Often a pet will be anxious, have a behavioral issue or even a health issue because of the energy they are absorbing from people around them. The Pet Balancing Spray contains flower essences and high vibrational crystal energies, Lavender Oil and blessed water. This can be sprayed around the pet (being careful not to spray in their eyes) or you can spray it on their bedding or the area they like to sleep.

REMEDIES FOR COMMON AILMENTS

For centuries essential oils have been used to cure many ailments, both physical and emotional. Here are some examples of uses:

- Sore Throat
- Flu Symptoms
- Ulcers and Infections
- Skin Irritations or Blemishes
- Dark Circles and Face Wrinkles
- Indigestion
- Headaches, Nausea
- Insomnia/Stress

- Ovaries/Menopause/
  Relationship Issues
- Issues with Love
- Aches and Pains
- Weight (over weight)/Diabetic
- For Pets
- Doing Healing on Others

Sore Throat

*Respiratory blend, Immune Support Blend,
Throat Soothe Blend, Oil of Oregano,
Manuka Honey, Colloidal Silver*

A sore throat starts as an energy imbalance
with communication. Meditate on who you
are not talking to or what you are holding
back. Sore Throat Blend, Respiratory Blend
and Immune Support Blend should all be
taken as soon as possible. They can be taken
in water or directly on the back of the throat.
Oil of Oregano can also be placed on the back
of the throat. These are all very strong, so
if you use them undiluted, which is great if
you can stand it, have a spoonful of Honey

(preferably Manuka Honey) ready to suck on and take away the initial burn. Colloidal Silver can be sprayed on the back of the throat, but you should not eat or drink or use any other oil for 15 minutes before and after the Colloidal Silver.

Flu Symptoms

Eucalyptus, Respiratory Blend, Immune Support Blend, Colloidal Silver, Ormus,

Immune Support Blend is the most important and should be taken as soon as possible. It should be taken orally. Either in a glass of water or directly under the tongue. Use 10 drops 2-3 times a day until the symptoms subside. Take Eucalyptus and Respiratory Blend in a personal diffuser (placing them in a pan of water with your head over the top and covered in a cloth). Colloidal Silver can be sprayed on the back of the throat, but you should not eat or drink or use any other oil for 15 minutes before and after the Colloidal Silver. Ormus can be taken orally as a supplement as well as additional vitamins C and B.

Ulcers and Infections

*Colloidal Silver, Immune Support
Blend, Frankincense*

Take Immune Support Blend and Colloidal
Silver daily as soon as possible. Immune
Support Blend is the most important and
should be taken as soon as possible. It should
be taken orally. Either in a glass of water or
directly under the tongue. Use 10 drops 2-3
times a day until the symptoms subside.
Spray the Colloidal Silver directly on the
ulcer or infection as well as at the back of
the throat, several times a day. You should
not eat or drink or use any other oil for 15
minutes before and after the Colloidal Silver
orally. So, use the Colloidal Silver apart from
the Immune Support. Also use a few drops
of Frankincense rubbing directly on the ulcer
several times a day.

Skin Irritations or Blemishes

Lavender Oil, Egyptian Oil

For dark marks or sun-spots rub a few drops
of Egyptian oil directly on the skin. It is said
to fade and lessen dark spots and wrinkles

and can be used daily as a face oil. For skin irritation, cuts, sores or rashes add Lavender Oil. If it is a large area or a sensitive area of the body you can dilute these oils in a massage oil first. If you feel it is infected, add Colloidal Silver orally and rub Frankincense also directly on the sore.

Dark Circles and Face Wrinkles

Egyptian Oil

Oil of Moringa Oliefera is the Egyptian oil known for rejuvenation. It is amazing for the face and skin. I use it directly as a face moisturizer and find it wonderful, especially for removing dark eye circles or blemishes. For dark marks or sunspots rub a few drops of Egyptian oil directly on the skin. It is said to fade and lessen dark spots and wrinkles. It can be used all over the body and is soft and soothing. To extend it you may want to add it to almond oil or coconut oil when used as an overall body moisturizer.

Indigestion

Peppermint, Ginger, Weight Loss blend

Take Peppermint and Weight Loss Blend orally. Either in a glass of water or directly under the tongue. Use 10 drops of each. You can add fresh ginger boiled in water or use ginger tea and add the oils to the ginger tea. Repeat after 30 minutes if symptoms have not subsided.

Headaches, Nausea

Peppermint

Rub about 5 drops of Peppermint on each of the temples and also on the third eye. Lie in a cool darkened room and try to relax if you are able. You can also put some drops of Peppermint in the palms of you hand and then inhale by cupping your hands over your face.

Insomnia/ stress

Lavender Oil, Rose-Geranium

Lavender Oil promotes relaxation and sleep. You can take a few drops orally. Also rub a few drops on your temples and around your chest and neck where you will be able to continually smell the aroma. It acts very good through inhaling. Put some drops in the palms of your hands and then cup your hands over your face to inhale. It is also great to put some on your pillow or head board, especially if you are using this to try to get to sleep. Adding to a few drops to a warm bath before bed is also a great way to relax the body. Lavender is a great oil to use added to massage oil or used in a wrap for relaxation. Rose-Geranium is another relaxing oil. It is fine to use the oils together. Rose-Geranium should be placed on the neck and shoulders where you can smell it. It is also great to add to a relaxing bath.

Ovaries/ Menopause/ Relationship Issues

Lavender Oil

Lavender Oil is known to balance the female hormones, especially estrogen. It is thought to stimulate the production of this hormone if it is needed and to balance the female hormone system. You can rub on your abdomen or you can ingest if you like the taste. Almost all issues in this area come from old relationship hurts that have not been fully resolved. Also meditate on letting go of hard feelings from old romantic relationships, or difficulties in current relationships.

Issues with Love

Lavender Oil, Rose-Geranium, Draw Love Spray, Third Eye Clear

Rub Lavender Oil on your sacral chakra (just under the naval) in a counter clockwise direction (from your right side to your left side). This will help to release old negative relationships, which you need to do before you can be open to a good positive relationship. A few drops of Rose-Geranium will bring out the feminine divine in a woman, bringing self confidence and attracting love. Spray Draw Love essence over your head in your aura to release blocks from your aura and draw your true love. Finally using third eye clear would help for you to be able to make clearer relationship decisions.

Aches and Pains

*Magnesium Oil, Peppermint Oil, John of
God ointment, Cadoka Oil, Filipino Oil*

Peppermint applied directly to the area of pain
as well as to the temples helps reduce the pain.
A few drops of Peppermint Oil could also be
taken orally either concentrated or in a glass
of water. If it is muscle, nerve or joint pain, use
Magnesium Oil by spraying on the soles of the
feet. The John of God ointment is wonderful
for areas such as backache or bruising. This
ointment is menthol based so should not be
used on sensitive areas of the body. Cadoka
Oil is wonderful for an overall body massage
(put a few drops in a massage oil or almond
oil). Sometimes pain is caused by negative
attachment, especially neck pain. For this use
the Filipino Oil on the back of the neck.

Weight (over weight)/ Diabetic

*Weight Loss Blend, All Clear Spray,
Filipino oil or blessed water/holy water
(if from being psychically sensitive).*

To lose weight as well as balance sugar
issues in the body, take a few drops of the

Weight Loss Blend orally, in a glass of water before each meal. These oils are believed to actually dissolve fat cells. Taken before meals it will also reduce the appetite. You can also use cinnamon to balance the blood sugar and to reduce the sugar from the blood. You can add cinnamon to water after eating to reduce the sugar in your blood.

We put on weight from absorbing other people's energy. If you are psychically-sensitive try also cleansing your aura. For this you can spray your aura with All Clear Spray and put a few drops of Filipino oil or Blessed Water on the back of your neck.

For Pets

Pet Balancing Spray, Lavender Oil, Frankincense Oil

Pets are very energetically connected to their "owners." So, in addition to "treating" your pet, make sure you work on the owner too. To calm and balance your pet you can spray Pet Balancing Spray around them or on their bed. They will also benefit as well as the humans to a diffuser with Lavender Oil to calm and sooth them. For arthritis, aches and pains, spray magnesium oils on the pads of their paws. For skin irritations use Lavender Oil directly on the skin irritation. For gum and teeth issues apply Frankincense directly on the gums.

DOING HEALING ON OTHERS

For the Healer

All Clear Spray, Filipino oil, Rose-Geranium, Third Eye, Colloidal Silver, Cakoda Oil – for the healer

When you are doing healing work on others it is good to protect yourself psychically. If you are psychically-sensitive try also cleansing your aura. For this you can spray your aura with All Clear Spray and put a few drops of Filipino oil or Blessed Water on the back of your neck. Rub a few drops of Cakoda Oil in the palms of your hands to allow energy to flow through you. A spray of Colloidal Silver in your mouth will help you to receive messages from spirit and stop your iron from being depleted. A few drops of Rose-Geranium on the third eye will enhance your mediumship. Rolling the Third Eye Clear on your third eye will open your third eye to be able to see more clairvoyant visions.

For the Client

Various Oils such as Rose-Geranium, Lavender, Frankincense and Third Eye Blend.

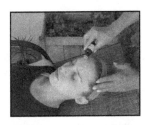

Oils and essences are wonderful to use on your clients during sessions such as Reiki and massage. Ask permission to use oils and essences on your client beforehand. Some oils are too strong to use concentrated on the body for massage and can be diluted into a body oil. Other oils can be directly used on the third eye and temples concentrated. You should talk to your client about what oils and essences you are using, and you can also muscle test their body.

OILS FOR PSYCHIC DEVELOPMENT

Some essential oils and blends can be used to open up your psychic abilities, manifest things and for psychic protection against negative forces. Here are some examples of uses:

- Psychic protection
- Increase intuition
- Manifest

Psychic Protection

*Frankincense, Filipino Oil or blessed water/
holy water, sage and Palos Santos crystals
black Tourmaline, All Clear Spray*

Before doing any psychic work, especially
working on others you need to protect
yourself. For this you can spray your aura
with All Clear Spray and put a few drops of
Filipino oil or Blessed Water on the back of
your neck.

Increase Intuition

*Rose-Geranium, Frankincense,
Third Eye Opening, Colloidal Silver
(clairaudience), Ormus, Moringa
Oliefera (if Egyptian influence)*

A spray of Colloidal Silver in your mouth will
help you to receive messages from spirit and
stop your iron from being depleted. A few
drops of Rose-Geranium on the third eye will
enhance your mediumship. Rolling the Third
Eye Clear on your third eye will open your
third eye to be able to see more clairvoyant
visions. If you are drawn to Egyptian Oil, this

may increase your connection to Egyptian spirit guides.

Manifest

Prosperity Spray, Frankincense

Spray Prosperity Spray in your aura, also in your handbag and or around your office. This is a combination of essences and oils known to draw abundance and success as well as confidence and strength. This spray helps to remove and cleanse any blocks of lack or other issues that are holding you back. It contains flower essences and high vibrational crystal energies and blessed water. Especially use this before an important meeting. Frankincense is also great for manifesting success. You can inhale it right before a meeting or place a few drops where you will be able to smell it.

OILS FOR CEREMONY & PRAYER

Rose-Geranium, Frankincense, All Clear Spray

Use Rose-Geranium, Frankincense on your altar in a burner or to anoint objects or use on your third eye during meditation. Use All Clear Spray around your aura and around your space for protection whenever doing any type of psychic work.

BATHS, WRAPS
AND OIL THERAPY

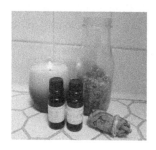

You can make your own soaking baths
or wraps with oils and create your own
mini ceremony.

Baths

To make the most out of an essential oil bath, make sure you have sufficient time to relax undisturbed. Set the scene for a perfect relaxing and meditating space. If you can do it safely, place candles by your tub. A white or purple candle as a protection candle with other candles for your purpose if you desire. Protect the room by spraying All Clear Spray in the corners of the room and around the tub. Run the bath water until it is nice and hot and full, then add the ingredients to your bath. Here are some essential oil recipes;

Relax Bath

10 drops Lavender Oil

10 drops Rose-Geranium Oil

¼ cup Almond Oil

Dried rose petals or rose buds (optional)

When the bath is ready, add the oils and mix in the bath water then add rose petals on the top. Perhaps you have some soothing music. Now relax and soak for 20-30 mins. This is great to do at night right before bed. After you get out of the bath and get into bed, spray Magnesium Oil on the soles of your feet for a really god night's sleep.

Detox/Cleanse Bath

Half cup salt (preferably Himalayan or black/charcoal salt)

Half cup Epsom salts (preferable unscented)

10 drops Eucalyptus Oil

5 drops Frankincense

¼ cup Almond Oil

1 cup holy water/blessed water

1-2 cups coconut water

Spray All Clear around the room or burn some sage and Palos Santos wood in the room.

Mix the salts and oils in a bowl first. In the tub, first massage the salt and oil mixture like a scrub on to your neck and shoulders and the soles of your feet. Then soak in the tub, allowing the salt mixture to now dissolve throughout the bath. Add holy water or blessed water, pour over your crown chakra (the top of your head). Now pour the coconut water over your crown chakra. Soak for 20-30 mins. Do not rinse the coconut water off your head if you can avoid it for 24 hours.

Increase Intuition Bath

Half cup Epsom salts (preferable unscented)

10 drops Rose-Geranium Oil

5 drops Egyptian Oil

5 drops Frankincense

Third Eye Opener

¼ cup Almond Oil

Place the Third Eye Oil over your third eye. When the bath is ready, add the rest of the oils and salt in the bath water. Now relax and soak for 20-30 mins.

Manifest/Success Bath

Prosperity Spray

Half cup salt (preferably Himalayan or black/charcoal salt)

Half cup Epsom salts (preferable unscented)

10 drops Eucalyptus Oil

5 drops Frankincense

¼ cup Almond Oil

Add a dark green candle to draw money

Spray the Prosperity Spray around the tub and around your aura. Mix the salts and oils in a bowl first. In the tub, first massage the salt and oil mixture like a scrub into your lower back. Then soak in the tub, allowing the salt mixture to now dissolve throughout the bath. Soak for 20-30 mins while you meditate on what you want to manifest.

Shower Scrubs

You can use these same recipes to make shower scrubs. Use salt as the scrub base for a detox shower scrub. For the other scrubs you may substitute sugar as the base instead of salt if you prefer. You may need to add more oil to make a scrub consistency.

Wraps

To make a wrap, you can follow the recipes but omit salt or sugar. You may need to add more almond oil. Mix the essential oils into the almond oil. Now massage the oil mixture all over your body.

To create a moist wrap, cover yourself in warm wet towels. Then a Mylar blanket, then additional dry towels on the outside. If you can now lie on a heating pad that would be great.

You can do this with your clothes on. Place the essential oils of your choice on your neck, shoulders, third eye and heart chakras. Lay on a heating pad. Wrap a Mylar blanket over the top to make a cocoon that keeps the heat in.

The heat from the wrap helps the essential oils to be inhaled and be absorbed into the skin.

TEST WITH YOUR ENERGY

We have talked about which oils and tinctures are suited for what issues and desires but ultimately it is the change in your energy and your results, that will determine success for you. Some have an inner instinct about oils, perhaps from ancient knowledge of past lives. You should always follow your inner guidance first.

Your body actually knows what your body needs and what would work for it. You can muscle test to see if the oil is the best one for you for the purpose. Sometimes you may be testing between one oil or another, but it could also be that you are asking your body to tell you how many drops to use or if a method of absorption is good for you.

The easiest way to ask your body if it "likes" an oil or tincture is to stand with your feet shoulder width apart and hold the bottle of oil over your heart. If your body "likes" the substance you will feel drawn towards it. If you body sways backwards, it doesn't need it, or it even may not like it. If you don't have the bottle physically to hold, you can just put your hand over your heart and say the name of the oil out loud.

You can ask a friend to muscle test you. To do this hold one hand out straight at shoulder height while holding the bottle of the oil in the other hand or anywhere on your body.

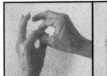

Loop Fingers   Fingers Lock   Fingers pull
               "Yes"   apart "No"

Another way to "muscle test" is to touch the tip of your first finger to the tip of your thumb to make a loop on each hand. Now interlock one loop to the other. In other words, lock the thumb and finger of one hand inside the thumb and finger on the other hand. Now ask for a "yes," and try to pull your two hands apart. If the answer is "yes," the loops should remain locked. Now ask for a "no" and repeat. With a "no" answer, the fingers and thumbs release and the grip falls apart easily. Now try asking about an oil. Either say the name out loud or place the bottle in your energy field (such as on your lap). If the fingers lock, your body likes this, if they release then your body doesn't need it.

If you get a "no" it could be that you have enough of this today or its not really that effective right now, but this could easily change a few days later and you can test again.

In a similar way you can ask; "Is three drops enough?" or "How should I use this. Would it be good to use this topically?" For the second question you may get a "yes" for both topically and orally. You could ask which would be best. An exception to this is don't ingest an oil that is not meant to be ingested, no matter what your energy test says.

At first your mind may overpower your subconscious and this may not work for you and it is best to just follow the normal guide lines. But keep practicing, after a while you can develop a good inner gage.

BOOKS BY
GAIL THACKRAY

*30 Days to Prosperity: A Workbook
to Manifest Abundance*

*How to Talk to Your Pets: Animal
Communication for Dogs,
Cats & Other Critters*

*Gail Thackray's Spiritual Journeys:
Visiting John of God*

*4 Reiki Certification Training Manuals:
levels I, II, III and Masters*

*4 Reiki Training DVDs: levels
I, II, III and Masters*

The Gift: Psychic Surgery in the Philippines

*What's Up with My Life? Finding
& Living Your Soul Purpose*

*Freaky Life Moments: A Medium's
Path to the Psychic World*

Mini Book Series

*How to Use a Pendulum: 9 Secrets
for Accurate Answers*

Gemstones for Love, Health & Abundance

Books are available on
Amazon or GailThackray.com

ABOUT THE
AUTHOR

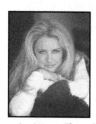

Gail Thackray has written about several metaphysical subjects, healing, developing psychic abilities and spirituality as well as about manifesting, soul-purpose and life missions. She also teaches workshops from time to time on Reiki, healing, manifesting, empowerment, past-lives and spirituality. Gail is the host of a documentary series, "Gail Thackray's Spiritual Journeys," where she travels to meet new-age leaders and experience places of great spiritual significance. Gail takes small groups on tours to spiritual places in Europe, Asia, South America as well as in the US. She teaches small retreats and takes people to visit healers such as John of God in Brazil. Join Gail on a life changing trip.

Gail prides herself as being down to earth and was entrenched in the business world when at age 40, she discovered she was a medium, able to connect with spirits on the other side. Gail was raised in Yorkshire, England and is now based in Los Angeles.

To find out more about Gail, her other books, her series and workshops, or to find out how you can visit her at a live event near you, please visit her website:

www.GailThackray.com

Go to

www.GailThackray.com/my-shop

to look at my essential oils